Sleep Well:

Tips and guidelines for quality sleep, established by the American Academy of Sleep Medicine

About the Author and the Lab:

The Sleep and Metabolism Lab (the SAM Lab) is interested in the role of sleep and circadian regulation in human health. Specifically, we study how sleep and circadian disruption impair physiological function, and whether improving the timing of behaviors such as sleep, exercise and eating can improve health and reduce disease risk.

The lab is directed by Dr. Josiane Broussard, PhD. Dr. Broussard is a leading authority in the field of sleep research, dedicated to unraveling the mysteries of sleep and its impact on human health and performance. With a passion for understanding the intricate workings of the human body, Dr. Broussard has devoted her career to exploring the relationship between sleep, circadian rhythms, and cardiometabolic health.

Dr. Broussard's pioneering work has been published in numerous peer-reviewed journals and has earned her recognition as a leading expert in the field. Throughout her career, Dr. Broussard has been committed to translating her research findings into practical strategies for improving sleep health and overall well-being. As a sought-after speaker and educator, she has shared her expertise with audiences around the world, empowering individuals to prioritize sleep and adopt healthier lifestyle habits.

In addition to her academic pursuits, Dr. Broussard is actively involved in public outreach and advocacy efforts aimed at raising awareness about the importance of sleep and the consequences of sleep and circadian disruption. Through her engaging writing and media appearances, she seeks to inspire others to take control of their sleep habits and unlock the transformative power of a good night's sleep. Check us out at https://www.broussardlab.com/

Table of Contents

Chapter 1: Maintain a Consistent Sleep Schedule
Go to bed and wake up at the same time every day, even on weekends. Consistency helps regulate your body's internal clock.

Chapter 2: Create a Relaxing Bedtime Routine
Establish calming rituals before bedtime, such as reading a book, taking a warm bath, or practicing relaxation techniques like deep breathing or meditation.

Chapter 3: Optimize Your Sleep Environment
Make sure your bedroom is conducive to sleep by keeping it dark, quiet, and cool. Invest in a comfortable mattress and pillows and consider using white noise machines or earplugs to block out disruptive sounds.

Chapter 4: Limit Exposure to Screens
Avoid electronic devices like smartphones, tablets, and computers before bedtime, as the blue light emitted can interfere with your body's production of melatonin, a hormone that helps regulate sleep.

Chapter 5: Watch Your Diet and Caffeine Intake
Avoid heavy meals, caffeine, and alcohol close to bedtime, as they can disrupt sleep. Instead, opt for light, easily digestible snacks if you're hungry before bed.

Chapter 6: Exercise Regularly
Engage in regular physical activity, but avoid vigorous exercise too close to bedtime, as it can stimulate your body and make it harder to fall asleep. Aim to finish exercising at least a few hours before bedtime.

Chapter 7: Manage Stress

Practice stress-reduction techniques such as mindfulness, yoga, or journaling to help calm your mind and prepare for sleep.

Chapter 8: Limit Naps

If you need to nap during the day, keep it short (20-30 minutes) and avoid napping too close to bedtime, as it can interfere with your nighttime sleep.

Chapter 9: Expose Yourself to Natural Light

Get exposure to natural sunlight during the day, especially in the morning, as it helps regulate your body's internal clock and promotes better sleep at night.

Chapter 10: Seek Professional Help if Needed

If you continue to experience sleep difficulties despite following these guidelines, consult with a healthcare professional or sleep specialist for further evaluation and treatment options.

Introduction

Introduction to Sleep: The Foundation of Health

In the hustle and bustle of modern life, amidst the endless to-do lists and constant distractions, sleep often takes a backseat. We push through fatigue, fueling ourselves with caffeine and adrenaline, unaware of the toll it takes on our health and well-being. But what if we told you that the key to vitality and productivity lies in something as simple (though not so simple to achieve) as a good night's sleep?

Welcome to "Sleep Well," a journey into the realm of sleep hygiene, guided by the comprehensive guidelines set forth by the American Academy of Sleep Medicine (AASM). Here, we will lay the groundwork for understanding the importance of sleep and the fundamental principles of sleep hygiene.

Sleep is not merely a luxury; it is a biological necessity, essential for our physical, mental, and emotional health. Yet, in today's fast-paced society, sleep deprivation has become endemic, with far-reaching consequences for individuals and society as a whole. From impaired cognitive function and mood disturbances to increased risk of chronic diseases, the effects of poor sleep are profound and pervasive.

Recognizing the urgency of the sleep crisis, the American Academy of Sleep Medicine crafted guidelines for sleep hygiene – a set of evidence-based practices aimed at optimizing sleep quality and quantity. These guidelines serve as a roadmap for navigating the complexities of sleep in the modern world, offering practical strategies to reclaim the restorative power of sleep.

At the heart of these guidelines lies the concept of consistency. Consistency in sleep schedules, bedtime routines, and sleep environments forms the cornerstone of healthy sleep habits. By aligning our behaviors with the natural rhythms of our body's internal clock, we can synchronize our sleep-wake cycles and promote a sense of balance and harmony.

But sleep hygiene extends beyond mere routine; it encompasses a holistic approach to sleep health. From managing stress and limiting screen time (easier said than done…) to optimizing our diet and physical activity, every aspect of our lifestyle plays a role in shaping our sleep patterns. By cultivating mindfulness and intentionality in our daily lives, we can create an environment that nurtures and supports restorative sleep.

As we embark on this journey, let us delve deep into the wisdom of The American Academy of Sleep Medicine, unraveling the mysteries of sleep and uncovering the secrets to a lifetime of restful nights and rejuvenating days. "Sleep Well" is more than just a book; it is a manifesto for reclaiming our right to sleep – a precious gift that holds the key to unlocking our full potential.

Chapter 1:

Maintain a Consistent Sleep Schedule
Go to bed and wake up at the same time every day, even on weekends. Consistency helps regulate your body's internal clock.

Chapter 1: Maintain a Consistent Sleep Schedule

Go to bed and wake up at the same time every day, even on weekends. Consistency helps regulate your body's internal clock.

In the symphony of sleep, consistency is the conductor that orchestrates harmony within our internal rhythms. Just as the rising sun marks the dawn of a new day, so too does a consistent sleep schedule signal the onset of restorative rest. Let us explore the importance of maintaining a consistent sleep schedule and its profound impact on our sleep health.

Imagine your body as a finely-tuned instrument, its melodies dictated by the cadence of your daily routines. By going to bed and waking up at the same time each day, you synchronize the intricate rhythms of your internal clocks, known as circadian rhythms. This internal timekeeping system regulates a myriad of physiological processes, from hormone secretion to body temperature, in anticipation of the cycles of day and night.

Consistency breeds predictability, allowing your body to anticipate and prepare for sleep. Consider the following scenario: Sophie, a diligent student, adheres to a strict sleep schedule, retiring to bed at 11:00 PM and rising at 7:00 AM each day. As a result of her disciplined approach, Sophie's body learns to release melatonin, the sleep-inducing hormone, at the appropriate times, facilitating a smooth transition into slumber. Conversely, her friend, let's call him Chad…lacks consistency in his sleep patterns, often staying up late on weekends and sleeping in on weekdays. Despite his efforts to compensate with caffeine, Chad finds himself groggy and irritable, his circadian rhythms thrown out of sync by erratic sleep-wake cycles.

Consistency extends beyond mere bedtime and wake time; it encompasses the entirety of your sleep routine. Establishing a bedtime ritual signals to your body that it is time to unwind and prepare for sleep. Similarly, creating a calming sleep environment, free from distractions and disruptions, fosters an atmosphere conducive to restful slumber.

But what about weekends, you may ask? While it may be tempting to indulge in staying up late and sleeping in on days off, straying too far from your regular sleep schedule too often can disrupt your body's internal clock. Instead, aim for consistency even on weekends, allowing for slight variations while maintaining the overall structure of your sleep routine. By honoring your body's need for regularity, you can reap the rewards of restorative sleep seven days a week. This may not always be possible, but you're playing the long game. If your sleep schedule starts to stray, think about getting it back on track. This is particularly important as we age and deep, restful sleep becomes even more elusive.

In the pursuit of optimal sleep health, consistency reigns supreme. By aligning your sleep-wake cycles with the natural rhythms of your body, you lay the foundation for restful nights and energized days. As we embrace the guiding principle of maintaining a consistent sleep schedule, let us embark on a journey of self-discovery, unlocking the transformative power of sleep one night at a time.

Notes/Reminders:

Chapter 2:

Create a Relaxing Bedtime Routine

Establish calming rituals before bedtime, such as reading a book, taking a warm bath, or practicing relaxation techniques like deep breathing or meditation.

Chapter 2: Create a Relaxing Bedtime Routine
Establish calming rituals before bedtime, such as reading a book, taking a warm bath, or practicing relaxation techniques like deep breathing or meditation.

As the day draws to a close and the world grows quiet, the stage is set for the nightly ritual of transition from wakefulness to rest. Let us explore the art of crafting a bedtime routine that nurtures tranquility and invites the embrace of peaceful sleep.

Picture this: The soft glow of lamplight casts a gentle warmth across the room as you settle into your favorite armchair, a cup of herbal tea cradled in your hands. The rhythmic melody of a soothing playlist fills the air, washing away the stresses of the day. This is your sanctuary, a sacred space carved out for relaxation and rejuvenation before bedtime.

A bedtime routine serves as a bridge between the demands of the day and the serenity of sleep, signaling to your body that it is time to unwind and prepare for rest. By engaging in calming activities that promote relaxation, you create a buffer zone between the busyness of life and the tranquility of sleep.

Consider the following elements of a relaxing bedtime routine:

Mindful Meditation: Take a few moments to quiet the mind and center yourself through mindfulness meditation. Close your eyes, focus on your breath, and allow yourself to let go of the worries and distractions of the day.

Gentle Stretching: Release tension and stiffness from your muscles with gentle stretching exercises. Pay particular attention to areas of tension, such as the neck, shoulders, and back, as you gradually ease into each stretch.

Reading: Escape into the pages of a good book or magazine, immersing yourself in a world of imagination and storytelling. Choose reading material that is light and uplifting, steering clear of stimulating or emotionally-charged content that may disrupt your ability to unwind.

Journaling: Reflect on the events of the day by jotting down your thoughts and feelings in a journal. Use this time to express gratitude, set intentions for the night and days ahead, or simply empty your mind of any lingering concerns or to-do list items.

Warm Bath: Indulge in the soothing warmth of a bath infused with essential oils or bath salts. Allow the water to envelop you in its embrace, melting away tension and inviting a sense of calm and relaxation.

Aromatherapy: Harness the power of scent to create a calming atmosphere in your bedroom. Experiment with essential oils such as lavender, chamomile, or bergamot, known for their calming and sleep-promoting properties.

By incorporating these elements into your bedtime routine, you create a sacred space for relaxation and renewal, paving the way for a restful night's sleep. As you embrace the art of crafting a relaxing bedtime ritual, may you find solace in the stillness of the night and awaken refreshed and renewed each morning.

Check out our favorite sleep-related items at
https://www.broussardlab.com/sleepswag

Notes/Reminders:

Chapter 3:

Optimize Your Sleep Environment

Make sure your bedroom is conducive to sleep by keeping it dark, quiet, and cool. Invest in a comfortable mattress and pillows and consider using white noise machines or earplugs to block out disruptive sounds.

Chapter 3: Optimize Your Sleep Environment
Make sure your bedroom is conducive to sleep by keeping it dark, quiet, and cool. Invest in a comfortable mattress and pillows and consider using white noise machines or earplugs to block out disruptive sounds.

Your sleep environment plays a crucial role in shaping the quality of your sleep. From the softness of your mattress to the gentle hum of ambient noise, every element contributes to the symphony of slumber. By optimizing your sleep environment, you create a haven of peace and comfort, free from the distractions and disruptions that can derail your journey to dreamland.

Consider the following guidelines for creating an optimal sleep environment:

Darkness: Darkness signals to your body that it is time to sleep by allowing the release of melatonin, a hormone that helps regulate sleep-wake cycles. Invest in blackout curtains or blinds to block out external light sources and create a cave-like atmosphere conducive to restful sleep.

Quiet: Silence is golden when it comes to sleep. Minimize noise disturbances by using earplugs, white noise machines, or soundproofing materials to create a peaceful sleep environment. If external noise is unavoidable, consider using a fan or soothing music to mask disruptive sounds.

Comfort: Your mattress and pillows play a pivotal role in determining the quality of your sleep. Choose a mattress and pillows that provide adequate support and comfort, allowing your body to relax fully into sleep. Experiment with different mattress firmness levels and pillow types to find the perfect combination for your needs.

Temperature: Keep your bedroom cool and comfortable to promote restful sleep. The ideal sleep temperature is typically between 60-67 degrees Fahrenheit (15-19 degrees Celsius). Use breathable bedding materials and adjust the thermostat as needed to maintain a comfortable sleep environment.

Clutter-Free: Clear the clutter from your bedroom to create a sense of calm and spaciousness. Remove electronic devices, work-related materials, and other distractions that can disrupt your ability to unwind and relax before bedtime.

Technology-Free Zone:* Banish electronic devices from the bedroom to minimize exposure to blue light, which can interfere with your body's natural sleep-wake cycles. Create a technology-free zone by removing TVs, smartphones, tablets, and computers from your sleep environment.

By implementing these guidelines, you transform your bedroom into a sanctuary of serenity – a sacred space dedicated to the pursuit of restful sleep. As you optimize your sleep environment, may you find solace in the stillness of the night and awaken refreshed and rejuvenated each morning, ready to embrace the day ahead.

*Creating a Technology-Free Zone in the bedroom is indeed easier said than done in today's digital age, where electronic devices have become ubiquitous and deeply integrated into our daily lives. Here are some reasons why implementing this particular guideline can be challenging:

Addiction and Habit: Many people have developed habits of using electronic devices before bedtime, whether it's scrolling through social media, watching videos, or responding to emails. These habits can become deeply ingrained, making it difficult to break the cycle of dependence on technology before sleep.

Entertainment and Relaxation: For some individuals, using electronic devices before bed is a form of relaxation or entertainment. They may rely on streaming services, gaming, or reading e-books as a way to unwind and destress after a long day. Breaking away from these activities can feel like sacrificing a source of comfort and enjoyment.

Work Demands: In today's hyper-connected world, many people feel compelled to stay connected to work at all times, including during evenings and weekends. The expectation of being reachable at any hour can blur the boundaries between work and personal life, making it challenging to disconnect from electronic devices, even in the bedroom.

Dependency on Alarm Clocks: While smartphones and other electronic devices often serve as alarm clocks for many people, relying on them for wake-up calls can make it tempting to keep them within arm's reach at night. Breaking this dependency may require finding alternative alarm solutions, such as analog alarm clocks or smart home devices placed outside the bedroom.

Social FOMO (Fear of Missing Out): The fear of missing out on social interactions, news updates, or important notifications can drive individuals to keep their smartphones or other devices nearby, even at bedtime. The constant stream of information and notifications can create a sense of urgency and anxiety, making it challenging to disconnect and unwind.

Despite these challenges, creating a Technology-Free Zone in the bedroom is not impossible. It often requires a conscious effort to establish new habits and boundaries around technology use, as well as finding alternative ways to relax and unwind before bedtime. Setting clear rules and boundaries for device use, establishing a relaxing bedtime routine, and gradually reducing screen time before bed can all help in transitioning to a technology-free sleep environment. Additionally, investing in alternative forms of entertainment and relaxation, such as reading physical books, practicing mindfulness, or engaging in calming activities, can make the transition smoother and more sustainable in the long run.

Check out our favorite items to help with relaxation at: https://www.broussardlab.com/sleepswag

Notes/Reminders:

Chapter 4:

Limit Exposure to Screens

Avoid electronic devices like smartphones, tablets, and computers before bedtime, as the blue light emitted can interfere with your body's production of melatonin, a hormone that helps regulate sleep.

Chapter 4: Limit Exposure to Screens

Avoid electronic devices like smartphones, tablets, and computers before bedtime, as the blue light emitted can interfere with your body's production of melatonin, a hormone that helps regulate sleep.

In today's digital age, screens have become an integral part of our daily lives, permeating nearly every aspect of our existence. From smartphones and tablets to laptops and televisions, electronic devices surround us, offering a constant stream of information and entertainment. Yet, as we immerse ourselves in the glow of our screens, we unwittingly disrupt the delicate balance of our sleep-wake cycles.

The blue light emitted by screens – known as high-energy visible (HEV) light – can interfere with our body's production of melatonin, the hormone that helps regulate sleep-wake cycles. Exposure to blue light in the evening hours can suppress melatonin secretion, making it harder to fall asleep and disrupting the quality of our sleep. Additionally, engaging with stimulating content on screens, such as scrolling through social media feeds or watching action-packed movies, can heighten arousal levels and delay the onset of sleep.

Consider the following scenarios:

Late-Night Scrolling: Cat, a busy PhD student, often finds herself scrolling through her smartphone in bed before falling asleep. Despite her best intentions to unwind, the endless stream of notifications and updates keeps her mind buzzing with activity, making it difficult to relax and drift off to sleep.

Screen Time Rituals: Raj, a medical student, has a nightly ritual of watching TV shows on his laptop before bed. While he enjoys the escapism and entertainment offered by his favorite series, he fails to realize the impact of screen exposure on his sleep quality. As a result, he struggles with insomnia and daytime fatigue, unable to break free from the cycle of screen dependence.

To mitigate the negative effects of screen exposure on sleep, the American Academy of Sleep Medicine recommends limiting screen time in the hours leading up to bedtime.

Here are some strategies to help you unplug and unwind before sleep:

Establish a Screen Curfew: Set a designated time each evening to power down electronic devices and disconnect from screens. Aim to limit screen time at least 1-2 hours before bedtime to allow your body to transition into a state of relaxation and prepare for sleep.

Create a Digital Detox Routine: Replace screen time with calming activities that promote relaxation, such as reading a physical book, coloring (check out our favorite coloring books), practicing meditation or yoga, or engaging in soothing music or nature sounds.

Use Blue Light Filters: If you must use screens before bedtime, consider using blue light filters or apps that adjust the color temperature of your devices to reduce exposure to stimulating blue light. Some devices also offer built-in "night mode" settings that automatically shift to warmer, less stimulating colors in the evening.

Designate a Charging Station Outside the Bedroom:
Create a designated charging station for your smartphone outside the bedroom. Choose a spot in a common area of your home, such as the living room or kitchen, where you can easily plug in your phone before bedtime. This not only prevents the temptation to check your phone in bed but also ensures that you start and end your day without the distraction of screens.

Indeed, limiting screen time in the bedroom, especially smartphone use, can be challenging given the addictive nature of these devices and their integral role in our daily lives. However, with some creativity and determination, it's entirely possible to establish boundaries and habits that promote a technology-free sleep environment.

Here are some even more creative ideas to limit smartphone use in the bedroom:

Set Up Night Mode or Do Not Disturb: Take advantage of the built-in features on your smartphone that can help reduce screen time in the bedroom. Enable night mode or do not disturb mode during the hours leading up to bedtime to minimize notifications and distractions. You can schedule these settings to activate automatically each evening to create a consistent routine.

Use a Physical Alarm Clock: Invest in a traditional alarm clock or a smart home device with alarm capabilities that can serve as an alternative to your smartphone. By relying on a separate alarm clock for wake-up calls, you eliminate the need to keep your phone within arm's reach at night, reducing the temptation to check it before bed or upon waking.

Create a Relaxation Corner: Transform a corner of your bedroom into a relaxation zone, free from electronic distractions. Fill this space with comfortable seating, soft lighting, and calming decor to encourage relaxation and mindfulness before bedtime. Dedicate this area for activities such as reading, journaling, or practicing relaxation techniques, fostering a screen-free environment conducive to restful sleep.

Create a Sleep-Friendly Playlist: Curate a playlist of calming music or nature sounds to listen to before bed. Choose tracks with slow tempos and soothing melodies to help quiet the mind and promote relaxation. Play your sleep-friendly playlist during your wind-down routine to create a peaceful ambiance in your home.

Try Audio-Based Entertainment: Explore audio-based entertainment options as alternatives to screen time. Listen to audiobooks, podcasts, or guided meditation sessions before bed. Close your eyes and allow yourself to immerse in the auditory experience, letting your imagination take you on a journey without the need for visual stimulation.

Embrace Old-School Games: Dust off board games, card games, or puzzles and make them a part of your evening routine. Gather your family or friends for a game night and enjoy screen-free social interactions. Engaging in these activities not only provides entertainment but also fosters meaningful connections with loved ones.

Practice Progressive Muscle Relaxation: Learn and practice progressive muscle relaxation (PMR) techniques as part of your bedtime routine. PMR involves systematically tensing and relaxing different muscle groups in your body to promote physical and mental relaxation. Incorporate PMR exercises into your nightly wind-down routine to release tension and prepare your body for sleep.

Create a Gratitude Journal: Start a gratitude journal to cultivate a positive mindset and promote relaxation before bed. Take a few minutes each night to write down things you're grateful for, moments of joy or kindness you experienced during the day, or reflections on what went well. Writing in your gratitude journal can help shift your focus away from screens and promote a sense of calm and contentment.

Use a Digital Lockbox: Consider using a digital lockbox or time-locking container to physically lock away your smartphone or other electronic devices during designated screen-free hours, such as before bedtime. Place your devices inside the lockbox and set a timer for when you want them to be unlocked. This physical barrier makes it more difficult to access your devices impulsively and encourages you to find alternative activities.

Implement a Reward System: Create a reward system for yourself where you earn points or rewards for every night that you successfully limit screen time before bed. Set up a jar or container where you can collect tokens or tickets as you achieve your goals. Once you accumulate a certain number of points, treat yourself to a reward, such as a relaxing bath, a favorite snack, or a movie night (screen time permitted, of course!).

Use a Screen Time Accountability Buddy: Partner up with a friend or family member and hold each other accountable for reducing screen time before bed. Check in with each other regularly to share progress, offer encouragement, and share tips for overcoming challenges. Knowing that someone else is counting on you can provide extra motivation to stick to your screen-free routine.

Turn Screen Time into a Game: Gamify the process of reducing screen time before bed by turning it into a game. Create a point system where you earn points for every minute you spend engaged in screen-free activities, such as reading, journaling, or practicing relaxation techniques. Set up challenges, levels, and rewards to keep yourself motivated and engaged.

By implementing these creative strategies, you can gradually reduce smartphone use in the bedroom and create a tranquil sleep environment conducive to restful sleep. Remember that consistency and perseverance are key, and it may take time to establish new habits and routines. With patience and determination, you can reclaim control over your screen habits and enjoy the benefits of a technology-free sanctuary for sleep.

Check out some of our favorite ways to promote relaxation before bedtime: https://www.broussardlab.com/sleepswag

Notes/Reminders:

Chapter 5:

Watch Your Diet and Caffeine Intake
Avoid heavy meals, caffeine, and alcohol close to bedtime, as they can disrupt sleep. Instead, opt for light, easily digestible snacks if you're hungry before bed.

Chapter 5: Watch Your Diet and Caffeine Intake
Avoid heavy meals, caffeine, and alcohol close to bedtime, as they can disrupt sleep. Instead, opt for light, easily digestible snacks if you're hungry before bed.

Your diet plays a crucial role in regulating various physiological processes, including sleep. The foods and beverages you consume throughout the day can influence your energy levels, mood, and sleep patterns. Similarly, caffeine, a stimulant found in many common foods and drinks, can have a significant impact on your ability to fall asleep and stay asleep.

Consider the following scenarios:

Evening Coffee Cravings: After a long day at work, Grissy finds herself craving a cup of coffee to perk up her energy levels. Despite knowing that caffeine can interfere with her sleep, she gives in to temptation and indulges in a latte from her favorite coffee shop. As a result, Grissy struggles to fall asleep later that night, tossing and turning in bed as the effects of caffeine linger in her system.

Late-Night Snacking: Levi often indulges in late-night snacks, particularly sugary or high-carbohydrate foods, as a way to satisfy his cravings and unwind before bed. However, he fails to realize that these foods can cause fluctuations in blood sugar levels and disrupt his body's natural sleep-wake cycles, leading to restless nights and fragmented sleep.

To optimize your sleep health, the American Academy of Sleep Medicine recommends watching your diet and caffeine intake, particularly in the hours leading up to bedtime.

Here are some guidelines to help you make mindful choices:

Limit Caffeine Intake: Caffeine is a powerful stimulant that can interfere with sleep by blocking the action of adenosine, a neurotransmitter that promotes relaxation and drowsiness. Aim to limit your caffeine intake, especially in the afternoon and evening hours, to minimize its impact on your sleep. Choose decaffeinated versions of your favorite beverages or opt for herbal tea or water.

Avoid Heavy Meals Before Bed: Consuming large, heavy meals close to bedtime can disrupt digestion and lead to discomfort, making it harder to fall asleep. Instead, opt for lighter, well-balanced meals that are easy to digest and include a combination of protein, healthy fats, and complex carbohydrates. Avoid spicy or acidic foods that can cause indigestion or heartburn, as well as foods high in sugar or refined carbohydrates that can cause fluctuations in blood sugar levels.

Watch Your Alcohol Consumption: While alcohol may initially make you feel sleepy, it can disrupt the quality of your sleep by interfering with REM (rapid eye movement) sleep, the stage of sleep associated with dreaming and cognitive restoration. Limit your alcohol consumption, particularly in the hours leading up to bedtime, and avoid using alcohol as a sleep aid.

Stay Hydrated: Dehydration can contribute to feelings of fatigue and lethargy, making it harder to fall asleep and stay asleep. Stay hydrated throughout the day by drinking plenty of water and other hydrating beverages. However, be mindful of consuming large quantities of fluids close to bedtime to avoid disruptions to your sleep due to frequent trips to the bathroom.

Mindful Eating Practices: Practice mindful eating by paying attention to your body's hunger and fullness cues and savoring each bite. Eat slowly and mindfully, focusing on the flavors, textures, and sensations of the food. Avoid distractions such as screens or work-related tasks while eating, as they can interfere with your ability to tune into your body's signals and lead to overeating or poor food choices.

By incorporating these dietary guidelines into your daily routine, you can nourish your body and mind, promote balanced energy levels, and create the optimal conditions for restorative sleep. As you make mindful choices about your diet and caffeine intake, may you find solace in the nourishing power of sleep and awaken each morning feeling refreshed, revitalized, and ready to embrace the day ahead.

Notes/Reminders:

Chapter 6:

Exercise Regularly
Engage in regular physical activity, but avoid vigorous exercise too close to bedtime, as it can stimulate your body and make it harder to fall asleep. Aim to finish exercising at least a few hours before bedtime.

Chapter 6: Exercise Regularly

Engage in regular physical activity, but avoid vigorous exercise too close to bedtime, as it can stimulate your body and make it harder to fall asleep. Aim to finish exercising at least a few hours before bedtime.

Physical activity is a natural and powerful sleep aid, influencing various aspects of sleep architecture and promoting overall sleep quality. Engaging in regular exercise can help regulate your body's internal clock, reduce stress and anxiety, and promote feelings of relaxation and well-being – all of which are essential for achieving restorative sleep.

Consider the following scenarios:

Morning Jogging Routine: Erin starts her day with a brisk morning jog around her neighborhood, soaking in the sights and sounds of nature as she moves her body. By engaging in physical activity early in the day, Erin sets the stage for optimal sleep later that night, as exercise helps regulate her circadian rhythm and boosts her mood and energy levels.

Evening Yoga Practice: Tyler unwinds after a long day at work with an evening yoga practice, focusing on gentle stretches and mindful breathing exercises to release tension and calm his mind. By incorporating yoga into his nightly routine, Tyler prepares his body and mind for restful sleep, as the relaxation-inducing effects of yoga promote a smooth transition into slumber.

To reap the benefits of exercise for sleep health, the American Academy of Sleep Medicine recommends engaging in regular physical activity, but timing and intensity are key factors to consider.

**Here are some guidelines to help you incorporate
exercise into your daily routine:**

Find What Works for You: Experiment with different types
of exercise to find activities that you enjoy and that fit your
lifestyle and fitness level. Whether it's walking, running,
cycling, swimming, or dancing, choose activities that you
find enjoyable and sustainable in the long term.

Prioritize Consistency: Aim for consistency in your exercise
routine by scheduling regular workouts throughout the
week. Establish a workout schedule that works for you,
whether it's in the morning, afternoon, or evening, and stick
to it as much as possible. Consistency is key to reaping the
sleep-promoting benefits of exercise.

Timing Is Everything: Pay attention to the timing of your
workouts, particularly in relation to bedtime. While regular
exercise can promote better sleep, exercising too close to
bedtime can have the opposite effect, as it may increase
arousal levels and make it harder to fall asleep. Aim to
finish your workouts at least a few hours before bedtime to
allow your body time to wind down and relax.

Moderation Is Key: Strive for a balanced approach to
exercise, incorporating a mix of cardiovascular, strength
training, and flexibility exercises into your routine. Avoid
overtraining or pushing yourself too hard, as excessive
physical exertion can lead to elevated stress levels and
disrupt sleep. Listen to your body and adjust the intensity
and duration of your workouts accordingly.

Pay Attention to Sleep Quality: Monitor how exercise
affects your sleep quality and make adjustments as
needed. Pay attention to how you feel after different types
of workouts and at different times of day. If you notice that

certain activities or timing interfere with your sleep, consider making modifications to your exercise routine to better support your sleep goals.

By incorporating regular exercise into your daily routine, you can enhance your overall sleep quality, boost your mood and energy levels, and enjoy a host of other health benefits. As you prioritize physical activity as a cornerstone of your sleep hygiene routine, may you discover the transformative power of movement and awaken each morning feeling refreshed, rejuvenated, and ready to seize the day.

Notes/Reminders:

Chapter 7:

Manage Stress

Practice stress-reduction techniques such as mindfulness, yoga, or journaling to help calm your mind and prepare for sleep.

Chapter 7: Manage Stress

Practice stress-reduction techniques such as mindfulness, yoga, or journaling to help calm your mind and prepare for sleep.

In the hustle and bustle of modern life, stress has become an ever-present companion, casting a shadow over our waking hours and infiltrating our dreams. Yet, in the sanctuary of sleep, we have the opportunity to find refuge from the chaos of the day and nurture our inner peace.

Stress is a natural and inevitable part of life, but chronic or excessive stress can take a toll on both our physical and mental well-being, disrupting our sleep patterns and compromising our overall sleep quality. Managing stress is essential for maintaining optimal sleep health and promoting a sense of balance and harmony in our lives.

Consider the following scenarios:

Work-related Stress: Lamya'a finds herself overwhelmed by the demands of her new job, constantly juggling deadlines, meetings, and responsibilities. As a result, she struggles with racing thoughts and worry, making it difficult to unwind and relax before bedtime. Despite her exhaustion, Lamya'a finds herself tossing and turning in bed, unable to find respite from the stressors of the day.

Relationship Strain: Oliver experiences tension and conflict in his personal relationships, leading to feelings of anxiety and unease. The strain in his relationships weighs heavily on his mind, causing him to ruminate and worry late into the night. As a result, Oliver finds himself trapped in a cycle of stress and sleeplessness, unable to break free from the grip of anxiety.

Here are some strategies to help you cultivate a sense of calm and tranquility in your life:

Practice Relaxation Techniques: Incorporate relaxation techniques into your daily routine to help reduce stress and promote relaxation. Techniques such as deep breathing exercises, progressive muscle relaxation, and guided imagery can help calm the mind and release tension from the body. Dedicate time each day to practice these techniques, particularly in the evening hours before bedtime, to prepare your body and mind for restful sleep.

Engage in Mindfulness Meditation: Embrace the practice of mindfulness meditation as a powerful tool for managing stress and promoting sleep. Mindfulness meditation involves focusing your attention on the present moment without judgment, allowing you to cultivate awareness and acceptance of your thoughts and feelings. Set aside time each day to practice mindfulness meditation, either through formal meditation sessions or informal practices such as mindful walking or eating.

Establish Boundaries: Set boundaries around work, technology use, and social obligations to create space for relaxation and self-care. Learn to say no to commitments that drain your energy and prioritize activities that nourish your soul and promote well-being. Create a bedtime routine that allows you to unwind and disconnect from the stresses of the day, setting the stage for restful sleep.

Seek Social Support: Lean on friends, family members, or support networks for emotional support and encouragement during times of stress. Share your thoughts and feelings with trusted individuals who can offer perspective, empathy, and guidance. Cultivate meaningful connections and prioritize quality time with loved ones to foster a sense of belonging and connection.

Engage in Physical Activity: Incorporate regular physical activity into your routine as a natural stress reliever and mood booster. Exercise releases endorphins, chemicals in the brain that act as natural painkillers and mood elevators, helping to reduce stress and promote feelings of well-being. Aim for at least 30 minutes of moderate-intensity exercise most days of the week, but avoid vigorous exercise close to bedtime, as it may interfere with sleep.

Practice Gratitude and Positivity: Cultivate an attitude of gratitude and positivity by focusing on the blessings and joys in your life, even during challenging times. Keep a gratitude journal or take time each day to reflect on the things you're thankful for, no matter how small. Shifting your focus from worries and stressors to moments of gratitude and positivity can help reduce anxiety and promote a sense of calmness and contentment.

By actively managing stress and prioritizing self-care, you can create the optimal conditions for restful sleep and overall well-being. As you embrace the practice of stress management, may you find solace in the quiet moments of the night and awaken each morning feeling refreshed, renewed, and ready to embrace the day with clarity and vitality.

Notes/Reminders:

Chapter 8:

Limit Naps
If you need to nap during the day, keep it short (20-30 minutes) and avoid napping too close to bedtime, as it can interfere with your nighttime sleep.

Chapter 8: Limit Naps
If you need to nap during the day, keep it short (20-30 minutes) and avoid napping too close to bedtime, as it can interfere with your nighttime sleep.

Naps, those brief respites from the demands of the day, hold the promise of instant rejuvenation and renewed energy. Yet, while a well-timed nap can provide a much-needed boost, excessive or poorly timed napping can wreak havoc on your sleep-wake cycle, leaving you feeling groggy and disoriented. Guided by the guidance of the American Academy of Sleep Medicine, let us explore the delicate balance of napping and discover how limiting naps can pave the way for more restful nights and vibrant days.

Napping is a common practice across cultures and has been associated with various benefits, including improved alertness, enhanced cognitive function, and reduced fatigue. However, when naps are taken too frequently, too long, or too close to bedtime, they can disrupt your natural sleep patterns and interfere with your ability to achieve restorative sleep at night.

Consider the following scenarios:

Afternoon Siesta: Laurel, feeling exhausted after a sleepless night, decides to take a long nap in the late afternoon to catch up on lost sleep. While she initially feels refreshed upon waking, Laurel finds herself struggling to fall asleep later that night, tossing and turning as her body struggles to adjust to an irregular sleep schedule.

Evening Power Nap: Sam, feeling sluggish after a heavy meal, decides to take a quick power nap in the early evening to recharge his energy levels. However, what was intended as a brief rest turns into a prolonged nap, leaving

Sam feeling disoriented and groggy when he wakes up. As a result, he struggles to fall asleep at his usual bedtime, further disrupting his sleep schedule.

Here are some guidelines to help you strike the right balance:

Keep Naps Short: Aim to keep your naps short and sweet, ideally lasting no longer than 20-30 minutes. Short naps can provide a quick energy boost without entering into deeper stages of sleep, making it easier to wake up feeling refreshed and alert. Avoid long naps, which can lead to sleep inertia – that groggy feeling you experience upon waking from deep sleep.

Time Your Naps Wisely: Pay attention to the timing of your naps and avoid napping too close to bedtime. Aim to take your nap earlier in the day, ideally in the late morning or early afternoon, to minimize its impact on your nighttime sleep. Napping too late in the day can interfere with your ability to fall asleep at night and disrupt your overall sleep schedule.

Create a Nap-Friendly Environment: Set the stage for successful napping by creating a comfortable and conducive environment. Choose a quiet, dimly lit space where you can relax and unwind without distractions. Use earplugs or white noise machines to block out external noise and consider using a sleep mask to block out light and signal to your body that it's time to rest.

Listen to Your Body: Pay attention to your body's signals and listen to your internal clock when determining whether to take a nap. If you're feeling genuinely tired and fatigued, a short nap may be just what you need to recharge your batteries. However, if you're feeling relatively alert and energetic, it may be best to forgo the nap and focus on staying active and engaged until bedtime.

Establish a Consistent Sleep Schedule: Maintain a consistent sleep schedule by going to bed and waking up at the same time every day, even on weekends. Consistency is key to regulating your body's internal clock and promoting healthy sleep patterns. By sticking to a regular sleep schedule, you reduce the need for daytime napping and ensure that you get the restorative sleep your body needs.

By limiting naps and paying attention to their timing and duration, you can strike the right balance between daytime rest and nighttime sleep, optimizing your overall sleep health and well-being. As you embrace the power of restraint and mindfulness in your napping habits, may you find harmony and balance in your sleep-wake cycle, awakening each morning feeling refreshed, revitalized, and ready to embrace the day with renewed energy and vitality.

Check out some of our favorite ways to nap:
https://www.broussardlab.com/sleepswag

Notes/Reminders:

Chapter 9:

Expose Yourself to Natural Light
Get exposure to natural sunlight during the day, especially in the morning, as it helps regulate your body's internal clock and promotes better sleep at night.

Chapter 9: Expose Yourself to Natural Light

Get exposure to natural sunlight during the day, especially in the morning, as it helps regulate your body's internal clock and promotes better sleep at night.

Light serves as the primary regulator of our internal biological clock, known as the circadian rhythm, which governs our sleep-wake cycles and numerous physiological processes. Exposure to natural light, particularly during the daytime, helps synchronize our circadian rhythm, promoting wakefulness and alertness during the day and restful sleep at night.

Consider the following scenarios:

Morning Sunlight: Maddie starts her day by opening the curtains and allowing natural sunlight to flood her bedroom. As she basks in the gentle morning light, her body receives a powerful signal to wake up and embrace the day. By exposing herself to natural light early in the morning, Maddie helps set her internal clock and establish a healthy sleep-wake cycle.

Outdoor Activities: Jack spends his weekends exploring the great outdoors, hiking through lush forests, and soaking up the sunshine. As he immerses himself in nature, Jack absorbs the natural light and fresh air, invigorating his body and mind. By engaging in outdoor activities during the day, Jack enhances his exposure to natural light and promotes better sleep quality at night.

Here are some strategies to help you harness the power of natural light for better sleep:

Start Your Day with Sunlight: Begin your day by exposing yourself to natural sunlight, preferably within the first hour of waking up. Open the curtains or step outside onto your balcony or patio to soak up the morning sunshine. If you live in a region with limited sunlight or cloudy weather, consider investing in a light therapy lamp or dawn simulator to mimic the effects of natural light indoors.

Spend Time Outdoors: Make a conscious effort to spend time outdoors during the day, whether it's going for a walk, gardening, or enjoying outdoor activities. Seek out natural environments with ample sunlight, such as parks, gardens, or waterfronts, and immerse yourself in the sights and sounds of nature. Even brief periods of outdoor exposure can have a positive impact on your mood, energy levels, and sleep quality.

Take Regular Sun Breaks: Incorporate short breaks outdoors throughout the day to refresh your body and mind with natural light. Step outside for a few minutes during your lunch break or coffee break or take a brief walk around the block to recharge your batteries. These mini sun breaks help maintain your exposure to natural light and reinforce your circadian rhythm.

Limit Artificial Light Exposure at Night: In the evening hours, minimize exposure to artificial light sources, particularly blue light emitted by electronic devices. Blue light can suppress the production of melatonin, the hormone that regulates sleep-wake cycles, making it harder to fall asleep and stay asleep. Dim the lights in your home and avoid screens at least an hour before bedtime to signal to your body that it's time to wind down and prepare for sleep.

Create a Sleep-Friendly Environment: Optimize your sleep environment by maximizing exposure to natural light during the day and minimizing exposure to artificial light at night.

Keep your bedroom dark, cool, and quiet to promote restful sleep, and use blackout curtains or eye masks to block out external light sources that may disrupt your sleep.

By embracing the light and prioritizing exposure to natural light throughout the day, you can synchronize your internal clock, regulate your sleep-wake cycles, and promote better sleep quality. As you immerse yourself in the gentle rhythms of nature, may you find solace in the warmth of the sun and awaken each morning feeling refreshed, revitalized, and ready to embrace the day with clarity and vitality.

Check out some of our favorite lights:
https://www.broussardlab.com/sleepswag

Notes/Reminders:

Chapter 10:

Seek Professional Help if Needed
If you continue to experience sleep difficulties despite following these guidelines, consult with a healthcare professional or sleep specialist for further evaluation and treatment options.

Chapter 10: Seek Professional Help if Needed

If you continue to experience sleep difficulties despite following these guidelines, consult with a healthcare professional or sleep specialist for further evaluation and treatment options.

In the pursuit of better sleep, there may come a time when self-help strategies and lifestyle changes alone are not enough to address persistent sleep problems. Although many sleep disturbances can be managed through self-care and healthy sleep habits, certain sleep disorders and medical conditions may require specialized evaluation and treatment by healthcare professionals. Recognizing the signs and symptoms of sleep disorders and knowing when to seek professional help is essential for addressing underlying issues and restoring restorative sleep.

Consider the following scenarios:

Chronic Insomnia: Despite implementing various self-help strategies and lifestyle changes, Heather continues to struggle with chronic insomnia, experiencing difficulty falling asleep or staying asleep on most nights. Despite her best efforts, Heather's sleep problems persist, negatively impacting her mood, energy levels, and daily functioning. Recognizing the need for specialized care, Heather decides to consult a sleep specialist for a comprehensive evaluation and personalized treatment plan.

Suspected Sleep Apnea: Dan, a middle-aged man, has been experiencing loud snoring, frequent awakenings, and daytime fatigue for several months. Concerned about his symptoms, Dan decides to undergo a sleep study, where he is diagnosed with obstructive sleep apnea (OSA), a common sleep disorder characterized by recurrent pauses in breathing during sleep. With the guidance of a sleep specialist, Dan explores treatment options such as continuous positive airway pressure (CPAP) therapy to manage his condition and improve his sleep quality.

To optimize your sleep health and address underlying sleep problems, the American Academy of Sleep Medicine recommends seeking professional help if needed, particularly for suspected sleep disorders or persistent sleep disturbances.

Here are some signs and symptoms that may indicate the need for professional evaluation:

Persistent Sleep Problems: If you experience persistent sleep problems, such as difficulty falling asleep, staying asleep, or waking up feeling unrefreshed, despite implementing self-help strategies and lifestyle changes, it may be time to seek professional help. A healthcare provider, such as a primary care physician or sleep specialist, can conduct a comprehensive evaluation to identify underlying factors contributing to your sleep difficulties and recommend appropriate treatment options.

Suspected Sleep Disorders: If you suspect that you may have a sleep disorder, such as sleep apnea, restless legs syndrome, or narcolepsy, it is important to seek professional evaluation and diagnosis. Sleep disorders can have significant implications for your health and well-being, impacting your sleep quality, daytime functioning, and overall quality of life. A sleep specialist can perform diagnostic tests, such as overnight sleep studies, to evaluate your sleep patterns and provide tailored treatment recommendations.

Daytime Symptoms: Pay attention to daytime symptoms that may indicate an underlying sleep disorder or medical condition, such as excessive daytime sleepiness, fatigue, irritability, difficulty concentrating, or mood disturbances. These symptoms can significantly impair your cognitive function, performance at work or school, and overall quality of life. Seeking professional help can help identify the underlying cause of your symptoms and facilitate timely intervention.

Risk Factors: Consider your individual risk factors for sleep disorders, such as age, gender, family history, and lifestyle factors. Certain populations, such as older adults, shift workers, and individuals with obesity or chronic medical conditions, may be at increased risk for sleep disorders and may benefit from proactive screening and evaluation by healthcare professionals.

If you suspect that you may have obstructive sleep apnea, it is important to seek professional evaluation and treatment promptly. Obstructive sleep apnea is a serious sleep disorder that can have significant implications for your health and well-being if left untreated. Common signs and symptoms of obstructive sleep apnea include:

- Loud or frequent snoring;
- Pauses in breathing during sleep;
- Gasping or choking sensations during sleep;
- Daytime fatigue or excessive daytime sleepiness;
- Morning headaches;
- Difficulty concentrating or memory problems;
- Irritability or mood disturbances;
- Decreased libido or sexual dysfunction.

If you experience any of these symptoms, or if you suspect that you may have obstructive sleep apnea, it is important to consult a healthcare professional for further evaluation. A sleep specialist can perform diagnostic tests, such as overnight sleep studies, to confirm the diagnosis and recommend appropriate treatment options.

Treatment for obstructive sleep apnea may include lifestyle modifications, such as weight loss or positional therapy, and medical interventions, such as continuous positive airway pressure (CPAP) therapy or oral appliance therapy. With timely intervention and appropriate treatment, individuals with obstructive sleep apnea can experience significant improvements in their sleep quality, daytime functioning, and overall quality of life.

By seeking professional help when needed and addressing underlying sleep problems, you can optimize your sleep health and enjoy the benefits of restorative sleep. As you embark on your journey to better sleep, may you find comfort and support in the guidance of healthcare professionals and awaken each morning feeling refreshed, revitalized, and ready to embrace the day with clarity and vitality.

Notes/Reminders: